PLEASE READ FIRST

The information and recipes provided in this 28-Day Detox Smoothie ebook are for educational and informational purposes only. The information in this ebook is not intended to be a substitute for professional medical advice, diagnosis, or treatment. Always seek the advice of your physician or other qualified healthcare provider with any questions you may have regarding a medical condition.

The recipes in this ebook are intended for individuals who are generally healthy and not pregnant, breastfeeding, or experiencing any medical conditions. The author is not responsible for any adverse effects or consequences that may result from the use or misuse of any of the information or recipes in this ebook.

It is important to note that this ebook is not a substitute for a balanced and varied diet, and should not be used as a long-term solution for weight loss or other health issues. It is recommended to consult with a registered dietitian or other qualified healthcare provider before starting any new dietary regimen, including the 28-Day Detox Smoothie program.

By downloading and using this ebook, you acknowledge that you have read this disclaimer and understand that the information provided is not a substitute for professional medical advice, diagnosis, or treatment. You also understand that I Dr.Maria Talton is not responsible for any adverse effects or consequences that may result from the use or misuse of the information or recipes in this ebook.

Table of CONTENT

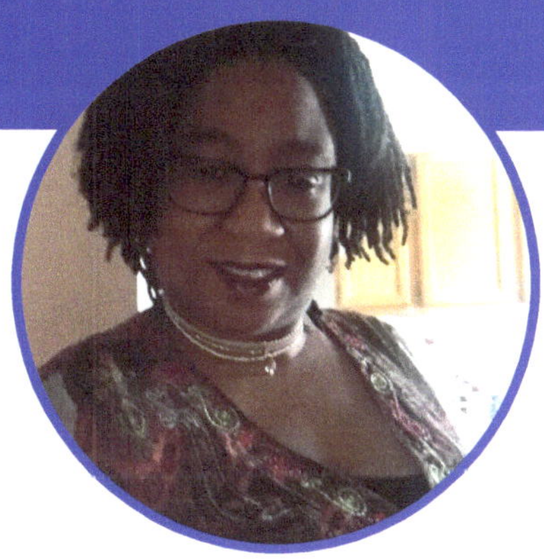

WELCOME!

Welcome to the 28-Day Detox Smoothie eBook!

I am thrilled to have you here and share my passion for healthy living through delicious smoothie recipes. This book is designed to help you jumpstart your journey towards a healthier and happier you.

Throughout this book, you will find 28 easy-to-follow recipes that use simple, whole food ingredients to help you detoxify your body, boost your energy levels, and improve your overall health. These smoothies are packed with vitamins, minerals, and antioxidants that your body needs to thrive.

I understand that starting a new diet or lifestyle can be overwhelming, which is why I have included a 28-day meal plan to help you stay on track and make the transition to a healthier lifestyle easier. The meal plans are customizable and can be adapted to fit your individual needs and preferences.

Please keep in mind that these smoothies are not a substitute for medical advice, and I recommend consulting with your healthcare provider before making any significant changes to your diet or lifestyle.

I hope that this book inspires you to incorporate healthy and delicious smoothies into your daily routine and helps you achieve your health and wellness goals. Cheers to a healthier you!

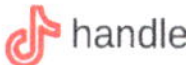 handle 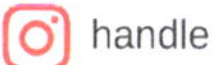 handle  handle  handle handle  handle

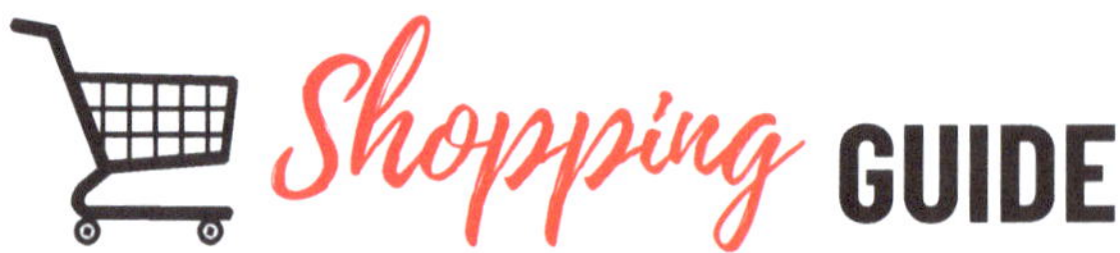

Shopping GUIDE

Welcome to the shopping guide page for my 40 Healthy Smoothie Recipes !I am excited to help you get started on your journey towards a healthier lifestyle. Smoothies are a great way to get in your daily dose of vitamins and minerals, and can be a quick and convenient meal or snack option. Before you get started with your smoothie-making, it's important to have the right ingredients on hand. Here are some tips for your smoothie shopping list:

FRESH AND FROZEN PRODUCE

The foundation of any smoothie is fresh or frozen fruits and vegetables. Look for fresh produce that is in season, or opt for frozen produce if fresh isn't available or if you want to reduce waste. Some great options include bananas, berries, mangoes, kale, spinach, and avocado.

LIQUID

To blend your smoothie, you'll need a liquid base. Water is the simplest option, but you can also use milk, almond milk, coconut milk, or fruit juice. If you're looking for a lower-calorie option, stick to water or unsweetened nut milk.

PROTEIN

Adding protein to your smoothie can help keep you feeling full and satisfied. Consider adding a scoop of protein powder, Greek yogurt, silken tofu, or nut butter.

HEALTHY FATS

Healthy fats can help your body absorb nutrients and keep you feeling full. Some great options include avocado, coconut oil, chia seeds, and flaxseed.

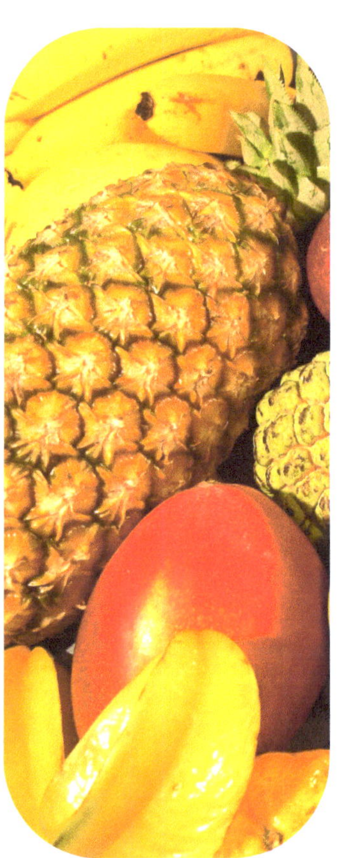

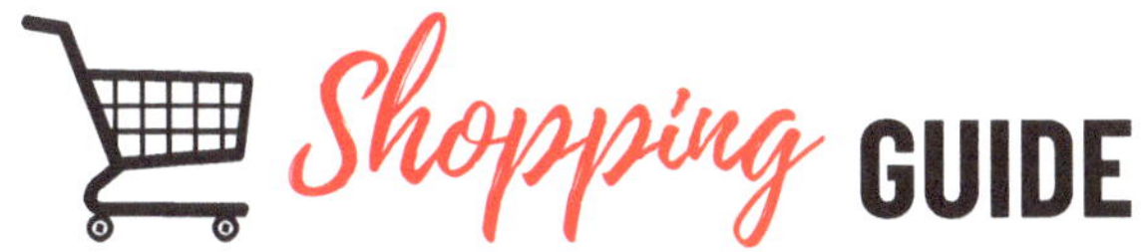

Shopping GUIDE

SWEETENERS

While you can sweeten your smoothie with fruits like bananas and dates, you may want to add a little extra sweetness. Consider using honey, maple syrup, or stevia as natural sweeteners.

EXTRAS

You can also add extras to your smoothie to boost its nutritional value. Consider adding superfoods like spirulina or maca powder, spices like cinnamon or ginger, or even a handful of leafy greens.

By following these tips, you'll be well on your way to creating delicious and nutritious smoothies with my 40 Healthy Smoothie Recipes . I hope this shopping guide helps you navigate the grocery store with ease and confidence. Happy blending!

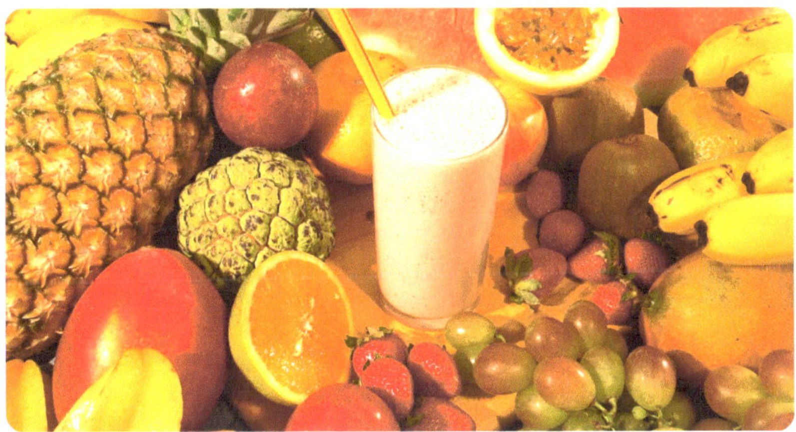

VEGETABLES AND FRUIT

Eating a variety of fruits and vegetables is essential for maintaining a healthy diet. They are low in calories, high in fiber, vitamins, minerals, and antioxidants, and can help with weight loss. When choosing fruits and vegetables for your meal plan, it is important to consider their nutritional value, freshness, and availability. Here are some tips on how to choose the best fruits and vegetables for your healthy meal plan:

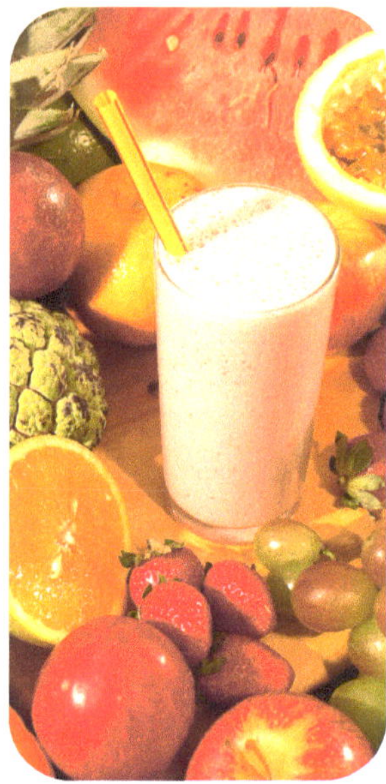

1. Choose a variety of colors: Different colors of fruits and vegetables offer different nutrients, so aim for a colorful mix. For example, dark leafy greens like kale or spinach are high in vitamin K, while orange fruits like oranges or apricots are high in vitamin C and beta-carotene.
2. Buy local and seasonal produce: Fruits and vegetables that are in season are often fresher and have more nutrients than those that are not. Try visiting your local farmer's market or joining a community-supported agriculture (CSA) program to get fresh, locally grown produce.
3. Look for freshness: Choose fruits and vegetables that are firm, brightly colored, and free of blemishes or bruises. Avoid produce that is wilted or has mold.
4. Consider frozen or canned options: While fresh produce is always ideal, frozen or canned options can be a convenient and cost-effective way to incorporate fruits and vegetables into your meal plan. Look for options without added sugars or preservatives.
5. Be mindful of portion sizes: While fruits and vegetables are healthy, it is important to watch portion sizes as they still contain calories. A serving size for most fruits and vegetables is about one cup, but some may be less, like berries or grapes.

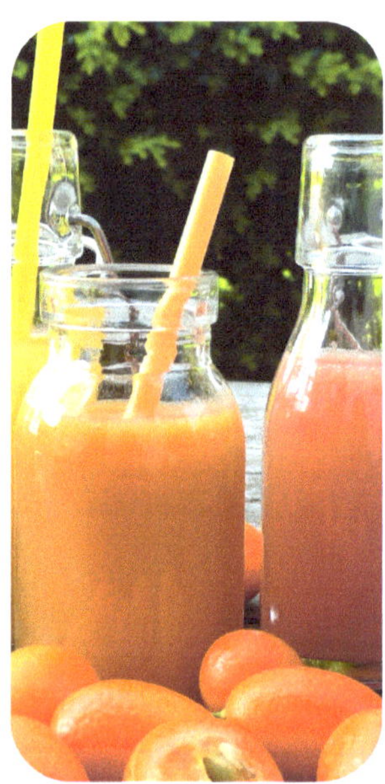

Incorporating fruits and vegetables into your meal plan can be easy and delicious. Try experimenting with new recipes and varieties to keep things interesting and enjoyable. Remember, the more fruits and vegetables you eat, the more benefits you will receive for your overall health and weight loss journey.

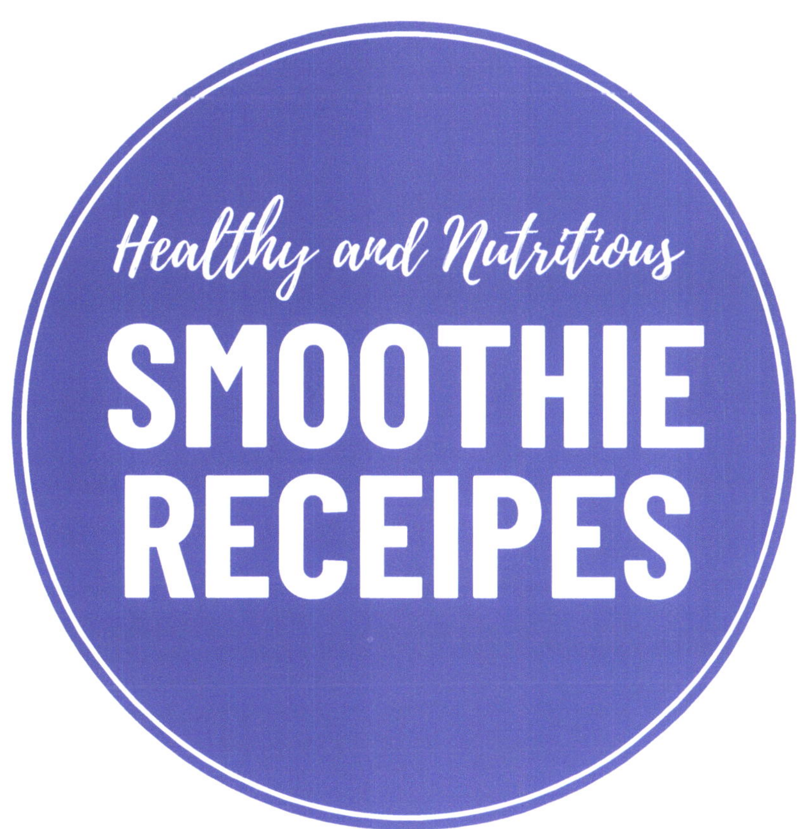

Healthy and Nutritious
SMOOTHIE
RECEIPES

INGREDIENTS

- 1 banana
- 1/2 cup almond milk
- 1/4 cup plain Greek yogurt
- 1 tbsp almond butter
- 1/2 tsp honey
- 1/4 tsp vanilla extract
- 1/2 cup ice cubes

INSTRUCTIONS

1. Peel and chop the banana into small pieces.
2. Add the banana, almond milk, Greek yogurt, almond butter, honey, vanilla extract, and ice cubes to a blender.
3. Blend on high speed until the mixture is smooth and creamy.
4. Pour the smoothie into a glass and enjoy!

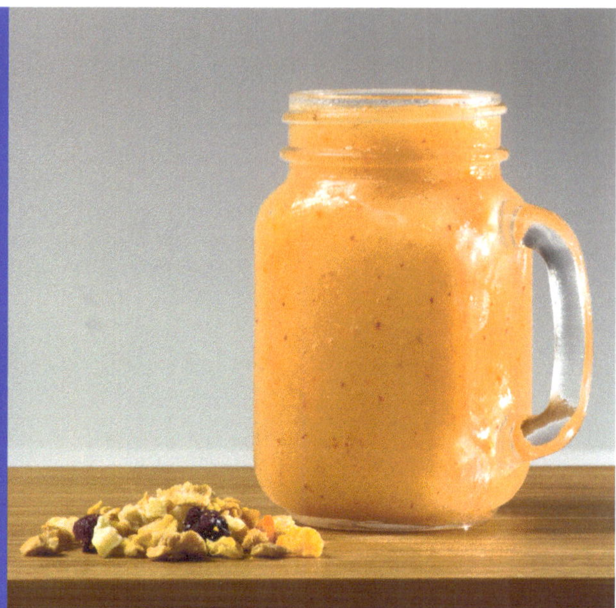

BANANA-ALMOND SMOOTHIE

 1 servings 　 5 minutes

This Banana-Almond Smoothie is a great way to start your day. It's packed with protein and healthy fats, which will keep you full and energized throughout the morning. The banana provides natural sweetness, while the almond butter adds a delicious nutty flavor. The addition of Greek yogurt adds a creamy texture and boosts the protein content even further. This smoothie is easy to make and can be enjoyed as a quick breakfast or a post-workout snack.

Nutrition Information (per serving):

- Calories: 230
- Protein: 10g
- Carbohydrates: 32g
- Fat: 9g

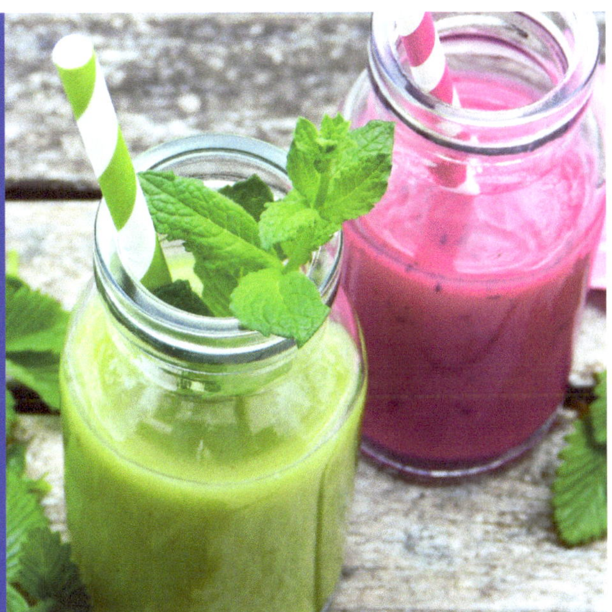

TROPICAL GREEN SMOOTHIE

 1 servings 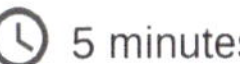 5 minutes

1. Add all the ingredients to a blender and blend until smooth.
2. If the smoothie is too thick, add more water until desired consistency is reached.
3. Taste and adjust sweetness and tartness with honey and lime juice as desired.

Nutrition Information (per serving):

- Calories: 240
- Protein: 4g
- Carbs: 54g
- Fat: 6g

- 1 ripe peach, peeled and pitted
- 1/2 ripe mango, peeled and pitted
- 1/2 cup plain Greek yogurt
- 1/2 cup unsweetened almond milk
- 1 tablespoon honey
- 1/2 teaspoon vanilla extract
- 1/2 cup ice

1. Cut the peach and mango into chunks and place them in a blender.
2. Add the Greek yogurt, almond milk, honey, vanilla extract, and ice to the blender.
3. Blend all the ingredients until smooth and creamy.
4. If the smoothie is too thick, add more almond milk or water to reach the desired consistency.
5. Pour the smoothie into a glass and serve.

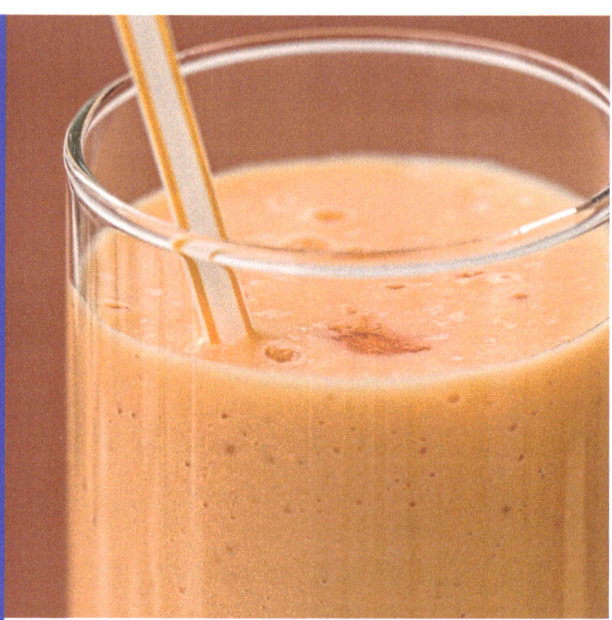

PEACH-MANGO SMOOTHIE

 1 servings 🕐 5 minutes

- This smoothie is packed with vitamins, minerals, and antioxidants from the fresh fruit, which can boost your immune system and improve your overall health.
- Greek yogurt provides a good source of protein, which can help keep you feeling full and satisfied.
- Unsweetened almond milk is low in calories and sugar compared to other types of milk, making it a healthier choice for this smoothie.

Nutrition Information (per serving):

- Calories: 260
- Protein: 11g
- Carbohydrates: 48g
- Fat: 4g

INGREDIENTS

- 1 cup chopped kale leaves
- 1 cup frozen pineapple chunks
- 1/2 banana
- 1/2 cup unsweetened almond milk
- 1/2 cup water
- 1 tsp honey (optional)

INSTRUCTIONS

1. Add all the ingredients into a blender.
2. Blend until smooth and creamy.
3. If the mixture is too thick, add more water or almond milk as needed.
4. Pour into a glass and enjoy!

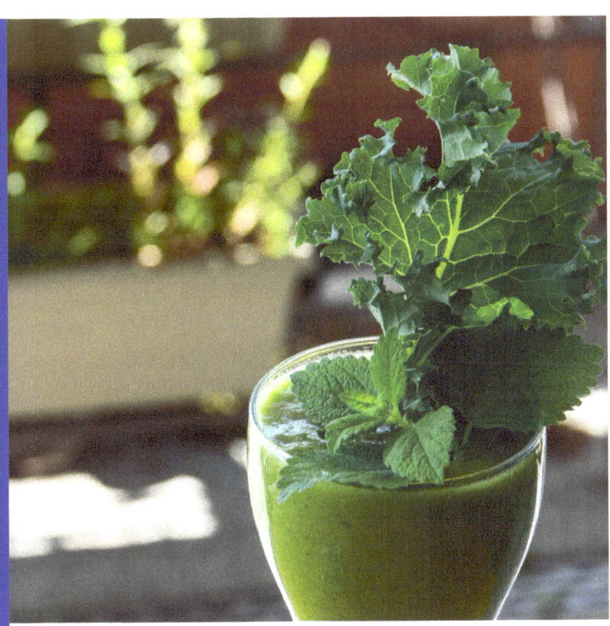

PINEAPPLE-KALE SMOOTHIE

🍴 1 servings 🕐 5 minutes

This smoothie is easy to make and perfect for a quick and healthy breakfast or snack. The kale provides plenty of vitamins and minerals, while the pineapple adds natural sweetness and a dose of vitamin C. The almond milk and banana add creaminess, and the honey (optional) adds a touch of sweetness. This smoothie is a great way to start your day or refuel after a workout, and at 300 calories, it's a satisfying and filling option.

Nutrition Information (per serving):
- Calories: 300
- Protein: 3 grams
- Carbs: 40 grams
- Fat: 2 grams

- 1/2 ripe avocado
- 1/2 cup frozen mango chunks
- 1/2 banana
- 1/2 cup unsweetened almond milk
- 1 tbsp honey
- 1/2 tsp vanilla extract

INSTRUCTIONS

1. Cut the avocado in half and remove the pit.
2. Add the avocado, frozen mango chunks, banana, almond milk, honey, and vanilla extract to a blender.
3. Blend until smooth.
4. Pour the smoothie into a glass and enjoy!

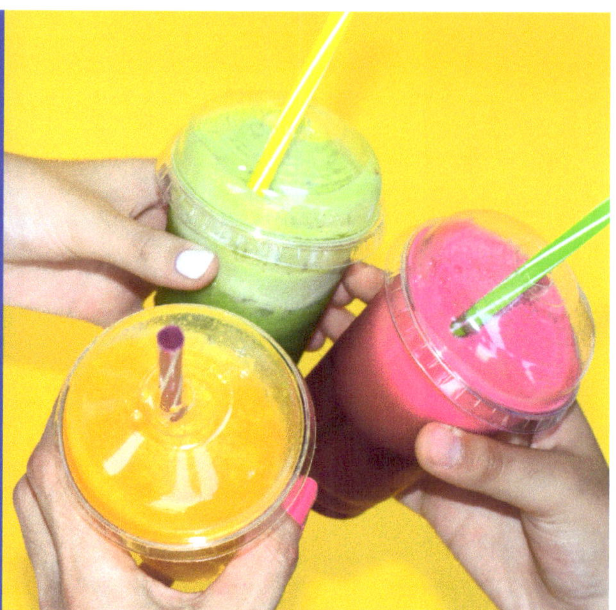

MANGO-AVOCADO SMOOTHIE

🍴 1 servings   🕐 5 minutes

This smoothie is very easy to make and offers a great balance of healthy fats, fiber, and natural sweetness from the mango and banana. The avocado adds a rich, creamy texture, while the almond milk provides a dairy-free source of calcium. Honey adds a touch of sweetness without any artificial flavors or colors. This smoothie is perfect for a quick and filling breakfast or a refreshing afternoon snack.

Nutrition Information (per serving):
- Calories: 320
- Protein: 4g
- Carbohydrates: 45g
- Fat: 15g

INGREDIENTS

- 2 cups watermelon chunks
- 1 small cucumber, peeled and chopped
- 1/2 cup plain Greek yogurt
- 1 tbsp honey
- 1 tbsp lime juice
- 1 cup ice cubes

INSTRUCTIONS

1. Add the watermelon, cucumber, Greek yogurt, honey, and lime juice to a blender.
2. Blend on high until the ingredients are smooth and well-combined.
3. Add the ice cubes and blend again until the smoothie is thick and icy.
4. Pour the smoothie into a glass and serve immediately.

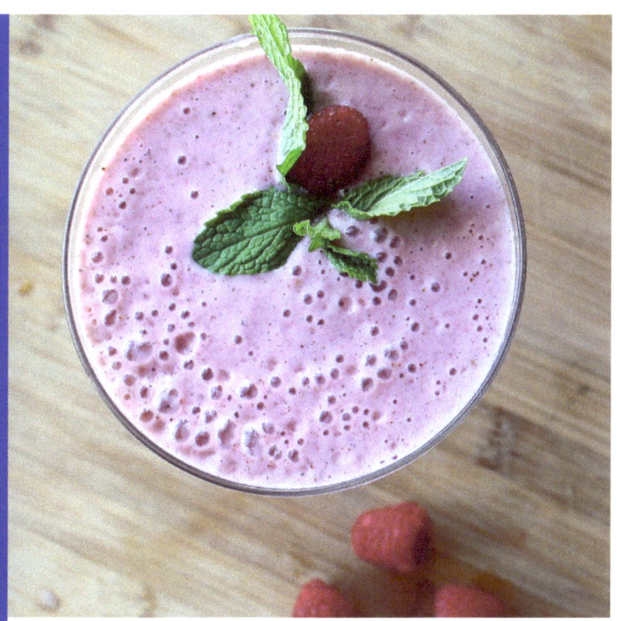

WATERMELON-CUCUMBER SMOOTHIE

🍴 1 servings   🕐 10 minutes

This smoothie is packed with hydrating watermelon and cucumber, as well as protein-rich Greek yogurt. The addition of honey and lime juice gives it a sweet-tart flavor that's refreshing and satisfying. This smoothie is easy to make and perfect for a hot summer day or a post-workout pick-me-up.

Nutrition Information (per serving):
- Calories: 340
- Protein: 13g
- Carbohydrates: 68g
- Fat: 2g

INGREDIENTS

- 1 medium carrot, chopped 1 medium
- apple, chopped 1 tsp fresh ginger, grated
- 1/2 cup unsweetened almond milk 1/2 cup
- water 1/2 tsp honey (optional) 1/2 tsp
- ground cinnamon
- (optional)

INSTRUCTIONS

1. Add the chopped carrot, chopped apple, and grated ginger to a blender.
2. Add the unsweetened almond milk and water to the blender.
3. If desired, add the honey and ground cinnamon.
4. Blend all the ingredients until smooth.
5. Serve immediately and enjoy!

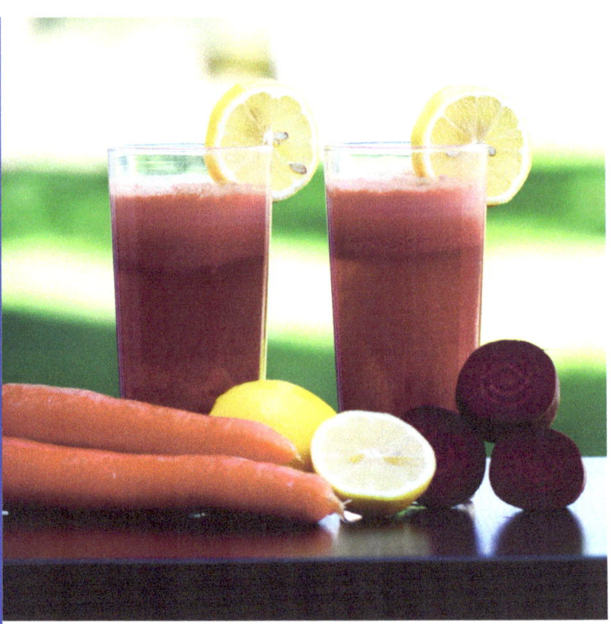

CARROT-APPLE-GINGER SMOOTHIE

🍴 1 servings   🕐 5 minutes

This recipe is easy to make and perfect for a quick and healthy breakfast or snack. Carrots are a great source of beta-carotene and fiber, while apples are packed with vitamins and antioxidants. Ginger has anti-inflammatory properties and can aid in digestion. The smoothie is low in calories and contains no added sugars, making it a great option for those looking for a healthy beverage.

Nutrition Information (per serving):
- Calories: 330
- Protein: 1g
- Carbs: 31g
- Fat: 1g

INGREDIENTS

- 1 cup frozen raspberries
- 1 banana
- 1/2 cup plain Greek yogurt
- 1/2 cup unsweetened almond milk
- 1 tbsp honey
- 1 tbsp lemon juice
- 1/2 tsp vanilla extract
- Ice cubes (optional)

INSTRUCTIONS

1. Add all the ingredients to a blender.
2. Blend until smooth and creamy, scraping down the sides as needed.
3. If the smoothie is too thick, add more almond milk or ice cubes as needed to reach your desired consistency.
4. Pour into a glass and serve immediately.

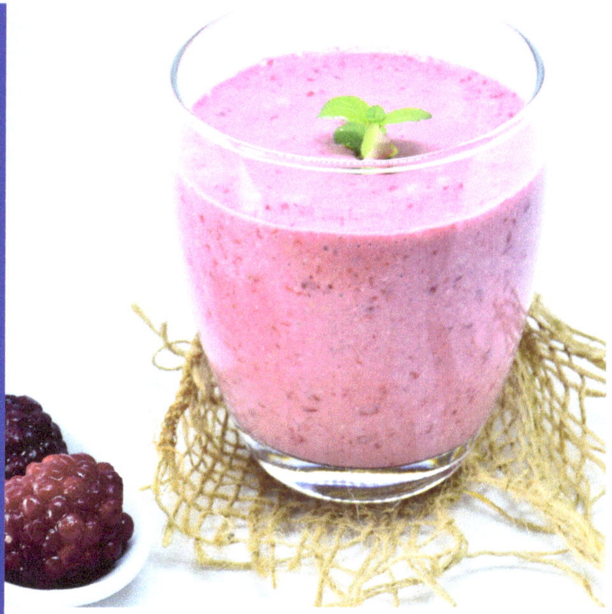

RASPBERRY-LEMON SMOOTHIE

🍴 1 servings   🕐 5 minutes

This smoothie is easy to make and provides a healthy dose of protein, carbs, and fat. It's packed with antioxidant-rich raspberries and vitamin C from the lemon juice. The Greek yogurt adds extra protein and creaminess, while the banana and honey provide natural sweetness. Overall, this smoothie is a delicious and refreshing way to start your day or refuel after a workout.

Nutrition Information (per serving):

- Calories: 350
- Protein: 11g
- Carbohydrates: 63g
- Fat: 7g

INGREDIENTS

- 1 cup fresh spinach leaves
- 1/2 cup frozen mixed berries (strawberries, raspberries, blueberries)
- 1/2 frozen banana
- 1/2 cup unsweetened almond milk
- 1/4 cup nonfat plain Greek yogurt
- 1 tsp honey
- 1/2 tsp vanilla extract
- 1/2 cup ice cubes

INSTRUCTIONS

1. Add spinach, mixed berries, frozen banana, almond milk, Greek yogurt, honey, and vanilla extract into a blender.
2. Blend on high speed until smooth and creamy.
3. Add ice cubes and blend again until smooth.
4. Pour into a glass and enjoy.

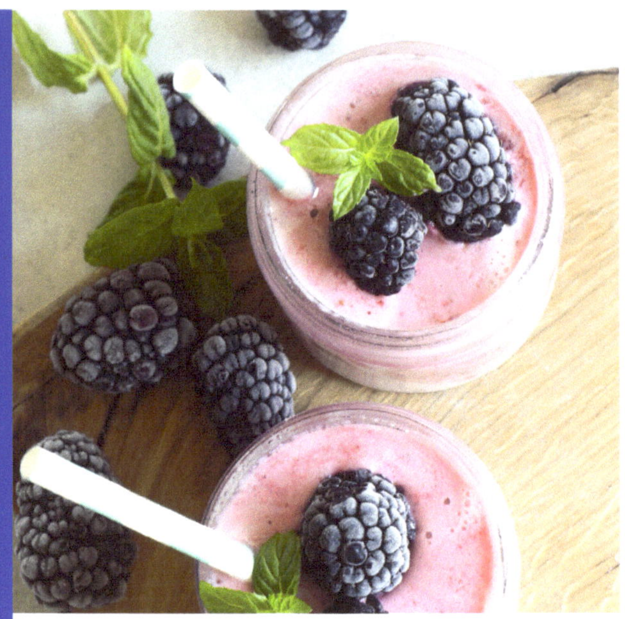

SPINACH-BERRY SMOOTHIE

1 servings 5 minutes

This smoothie is a great source of fiber, antioxidants, and vitamins from the spinach and mixed berries. Greek yogurt adds protein, while almond milk provides a creamy texture without adding extra calories. The honey and vanilla extract give it a touch of sweetness without any added sugars.

Nutrition Information (per serving):
- Calories: 360
- Protein: 20g
- Carbohydrates: 62g
- Fat: 5g

INGREDIENTS

- 1 cup frozen cherries
- 1/2 cup vanilla Greek yogurt 1/2 cup
- unsweetened almond milk 1/2 teaspoon
- vanilla extract 1 tablespoon honey
-

INSTRUCTIONS

1. Add all ingredients to a blender.
2. Blend until smooth.
3. Pour into a glass and enjoy!

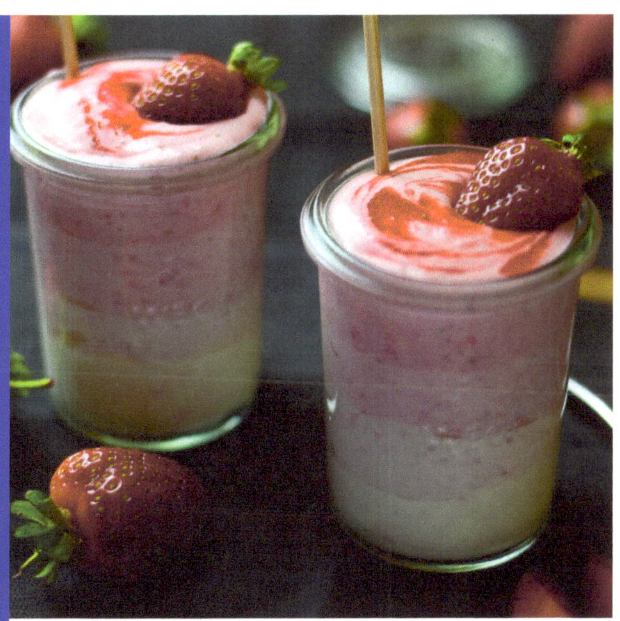

CHERRY-VANILLA SMOOTHIE

🍴 1 servings   🕐 5 minutes

This smoothie is a delicious way to enjoy the health benefits of cherries, which are rich in antioxidants and anti-inflammatory compounds that can help reduce inflammation and improve heart health. The Greek yogurt provides a good source of protein and calcium, while the almond milk adds extra vitamins and minerals. The vanilla extract and honey add a touch of sweetness and flavor to the smoothie.

Nutrition Information (per serving):
- Calories: 370
- Protein: 19g
- Carbohydrates: 66g
- Fat: 4g

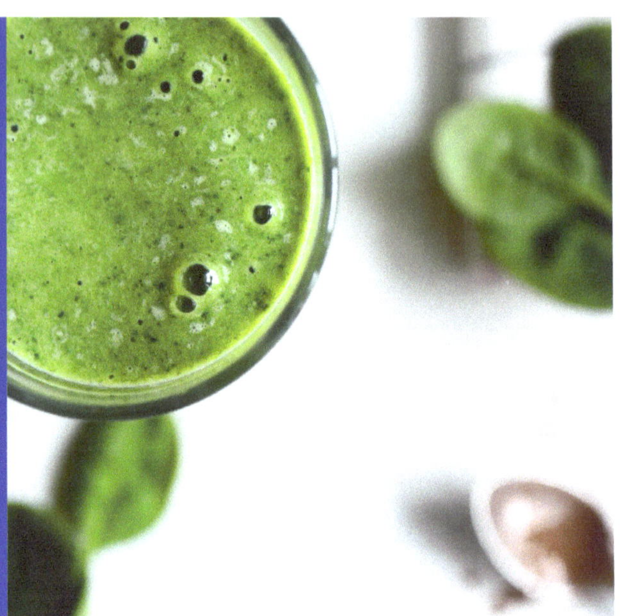

INGREDIENTS

- 1 ripe peach, peeled and sliced
- 1/2 cup brewed and cooled green tea
- 1/2 cup plain Greek yogurt
- 1/2 cup spinach leaves
- 1 tbsp honey
- 1/2 tsp grated ginger
- 1/2 cup ice cubes

INSTRUCTIONS

1. Brew green tea and let it cool down to room temperature.
2. Add all the ingredients into a blender and blend until smooth.
3. Pour the smoothie into a glass and enjoy!

GREEN TEA-PEACH SMOOTHIE

🍴 1 servings   🕐 5 minutes

This smoothie is packed with antioxidants from green tea, peaches, and spinach. Green tea also contains caffeine, which can help increase alertness and improve cognitive function. The Greek yogurt adds protein to help keep you full and satisfied, and the honey adds natural sweetness. The ginger can also help with digestion and reduce inflammation.

Nutrition Information (per serving):

- Calories: 380
- Protein: 19g
- Carbs: 56g
- Fat: 6g

INGREDIENTS

- 1 medium banana, sliced
- 1/2 cup frozen blueberries
- 1/2 cup unsweetened almond milk
- 1/2 cup plain Greek yogurt
- 1/4 cup rolled oats
- 1 tsp honey
- 1/2 tsp vanilla extract

INSTRUCTIONS

1. Add all of the ingredients to a blender.
2. Blend until smooth and creamy, adding more almond milk if necessary to reach your desired consistency.
3. Pour into a glass and enjoy!

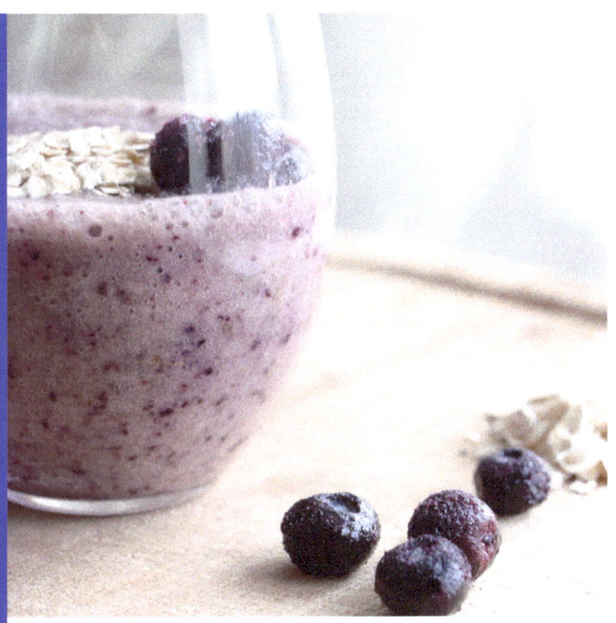

BLUEBERRY-BANANA-OATMEAL SMOOTHIE

🍴 1 servings 🕐 5 minutes

This smoothie is relatively easy to make and is a great option for breakfast or as a post-workout snack. It's packed with protein, fiber, and antioxidants from the blueberries, and the oats provide complex carbohydrates for sustained energy. The banana adds natural sweetness, while the Greek yogurt provides a creamy texture and additional protein.

Nutrition Information (per serving):
- Calories: 390
- Protein: 19g
- Carbs: 64g
- Fat: 5g

INGREDIENTS

- 1 ripe banana
- 1 tablespoon unsweetened cocoa powder
- 1/2 cup unsweetened almond milk
- 1/2 cup plain Greek yogurt
- 1/2 teaspoon vanilla extract
- 1/2 cup ice cubes

INSTRUCTIONS

1. Peel the banana and slice it into small pieces.
2. Add the banana, unsweetened cocoa powder, almond milk, Greek yogurt, vanilla extract, and ice cubes into a blender.
3. Blend all the ingredients until smooth and creamy.
4. If the mixture is too thick, add a little more almond milk until desired consistency is achieved.
5. Pour the smoothie into a glass and enjoy immediately.

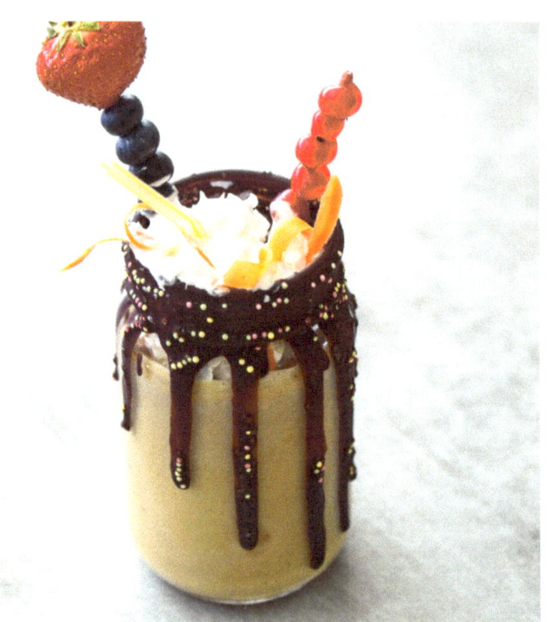

CHOCOLATE-BANANA SMOOTHIE

🍴 1 servings   🕐 5 minutes

This smoothie is a great way to indulge in a chocolatey treat while still getting a good dose of protein from the Greek yogurt. The banana also adds a natural sweetness and fiber to the smoothie, making it a healthier option than traditional chocolate milkshakes or smoothies. Additionally, the unsweetened cocoa powder contains antioxidants that may help improve heart health and lower blood pressure.

Nutrition Information (per serving):
- Calories: 410
- Protein: 29g
- Carbohydrates: 56g
- Fat: 8g

INGREDIENTS

- 1 medium-sized banana, frozen
- 1 cup brewed coffee, cooled
- 1/2 cup milk (you can use any type of milk)
- 1 tablespoon honey or sweetener of your choice
- 1/2 teaspoon vanilla extract
- 1/2 cup ice cubes

INSTRUCTIONS

1. Brew a cup of coffee and let it cool down to room temperature.
2. Peel the banana and cut it into small pieces.
3. In a blender, combine the cooled coffee, milk, frozen banana, honey, vanilla extract, and ice cubes.
4. Blend everything until smooth and creamy.
5. Pour the smoothie into a glass and serve immediately.

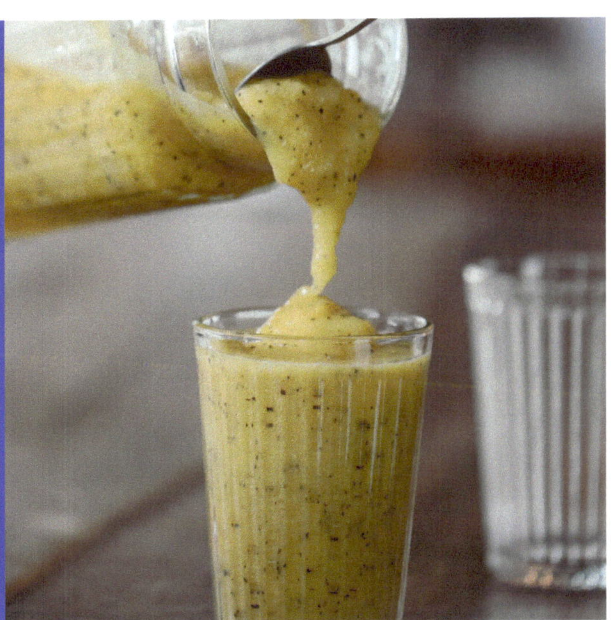

COFFEE-BANANA SMOOTHIE

🍴 1 servings 🕐 10 minutes

This coffee-banana smoothie is a delicious and energizing way to start your day. It's rich in potassium and antioxidants from the banana and the coffee, which can help improve heart health and protect against chronic diseases. Additionally, the caffeine in the coffee can provide a temporary boost in alertness and mental focus.

Nutrition Information (per serving):
- Calories: 420
- Protein: 7g
- Carbohydrates: 75g
- Fat: 11g

- 1 cup chopped mango
- 1/2 banana
- 1 cup spinach
- 1/2 cup unsweetened almond milk
- 1 tbsp honey
- 1 tbsp lime juice

INSTRUCTIONS

1. In a blender, add chopped mango, banana, spinach, almond milk, honey, and lime juice.
2. Blend until smooth and creamy.
3. If the smoothie is too thick, add a bit more almond milk or water.
4. Pour the smoothie into a glass and enjoy!

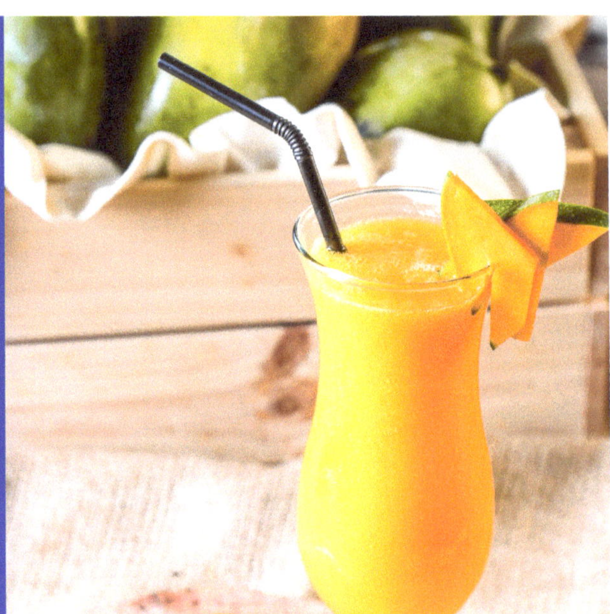

GREEN MANGO SMOOTHIE

🍴 1 servings   🕐 5 minutes

This smoothie is easy to make and has several health benefits. Mangoes are rich in vitamins and minerals, including vitamin C and folate, while spinach is a great source of iron and antioxidants. Banana provides additional fiber and sweetness, while the lime juice adds a tart and refreshing taste. The smoothie is naturally sweetened with honey and contains unsweetened almond milk, making it a great dairy-free option.

Nutrition Information (per serving):

- Calories: 440
- Protein: 4g
- Carbs: 92g
- Fat: 4g

- 1 ripe banana
- 1/2 cup rolled oats
- 1 cup unsweetened almond milk
- 1/2 tsp cinnamon
- 1 tsp honey (optional)
- 1/2 cup ice cubes

INSTRUCTIONS

1. Start by adding the rolled oats to a blender and blend until they are finely ground.
2. Add the banana, almond milk, cinnamon, honey (if using), and ice cubes to the blender.
3. Blend until smooth and creamy.
4. If the mixture is too thick, you can add more almond milk or water to thin it out to your liking.
5. Pour the smoothie into a glass and enjoy!

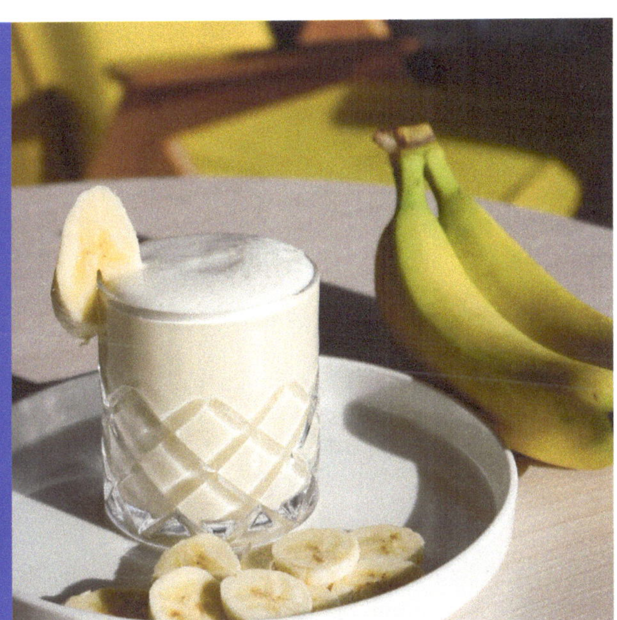

BANANA-OATMEAL SMOOTHIE

🍴 1 servings 🕐 5 minutes

This recipe is quite easy to make, and it's perfect for a quick breakfast or snack. The combination of banana and oatmeal makes it a filling and satisfying drink that will keep you full for longer. The cinnamon adds a nice warm flavor, while the honey (if using) provides a touch of sweetness. This smoothie is also a good source of fiber and plant-based protein, making it a healthy and nutritious option.

Nutrition Information (per serving):

- Calories: 450
- Protein: 9g
- Carbs: 78g
- Fat: 11g

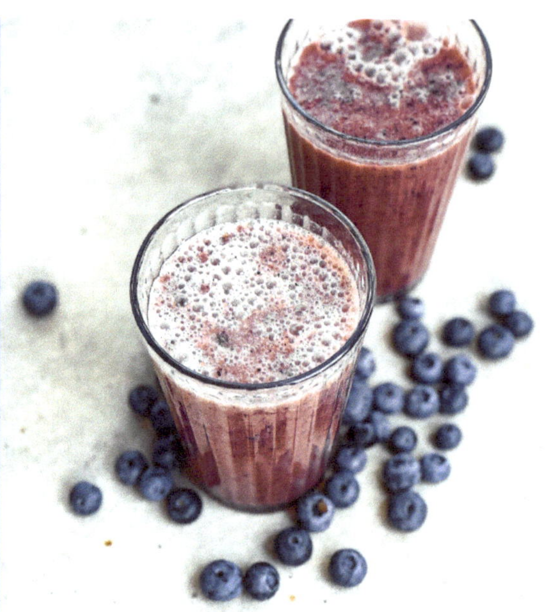

BLUEBERRY-AVOCADO SMOOTHIE

 1 servings   5 minutes

This smoothie is easy to make and provides numerous health benefits. Avocado is a great source of healthy fats and fiber, while blueberries are packed with antioxidants and other nutrients. The Greek yogurt adds protein and creaminess, while the honey and vanilla extract provide natural sweetness. Overall, this smoothie is a tasty and nutritious way to start your day or refuel after a workout.

Nutrition Information (per serving):
- Calories: 460
- Protein: 8g
- Carbs: 55g
- Fat: 26g

INGREDIENTS

- 1 ripe peach, peeled and pitted
- 1 small carrot, peeled and chopped
- 1/2 cup of unsweetened almond milk
- 1/2 cup of plain Greek yogurt
- 1 tablespoon of honey
- 1/4 teaspoon of ground ginger
- 1 cup of ice cubes

INSTRUCTIONS

1. Combine the chopped peach, chopped carrot, almond milk, Greek yogurt, honey, and ginger in a blender.
2. Add the ice cubes to the blender and blend until smooth.
3. If the smoothie is too thick, add more almond milk or water until you reach the desired consistency.
4. Pour the smoothie into a glass and enjoy immediately.

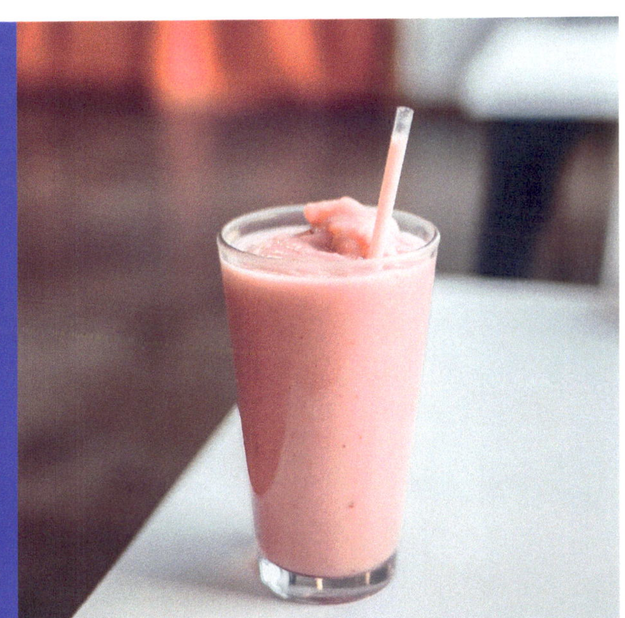

PEACH-CARROT SMOOTHIE

🍴 1 servings 🕐 5 minutes

This Peach-Carrot Smoothie is packed with vitamins and minerals. Peaches are a great source of vitamin C, while carrots are high in vitamin A. Additionally, the Greek yogurt provides protein, which can help you feel full for longer. The smoothie is sweetened with honey, which adds a touch of sweetness without any refined sugars. This smoothie is relatively easy to make and is a great option for a quick breakfast or post-workout snack.

Nutrition Information (per serving):

- Calories: 480
- Protein: 18g
- Carbs: 78g
- Fat: 4g

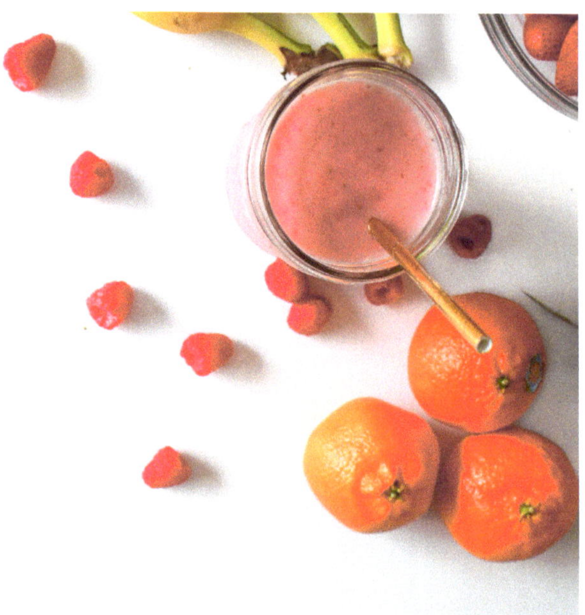

RASPBERRY-POMEGRANATE SMOOTHIE

🍴 1 servings   🕐 5 minutes

This recipe is easy to make and packed with antioxidants from the raspberries and pomegranate juice. The Greek yogurt and almond milk provide protein and calcium, while the banana adds natural sweetness and potassium. The smoothie is also vegetarian and gluten-free.

Nutrition Information (per serving):
- Calories: 500
- Protein: 12g
- Carbohydrates: 65g
- Fat: 5g

- 1 kiwi, peeled and chopped
- 1 cup strawberries, hulled and sliced
- 1/2 cup unsweetened almond milk
- 1/2 cup plain Greek yogurt
- 1/2 tsp honey (optional)
- 1/2 cup ice cubes

1. In a blender, add the chopped kiwi, sliced strawberries, almond milk, Greek yogurt, and honey (if using).
2. Blend the ingredients together until smooth.
3. Add the ice cubes and blend again until smooth and frothy.
4. Pour the smoothie into a glass and serve immediately.

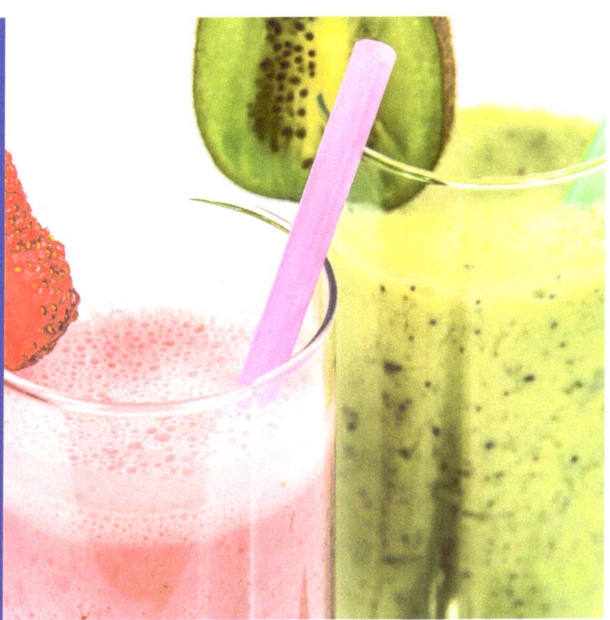

KIWI-STRAWBERRY SMOOTHIE

🍴 1 servings   🕐 5 minutes

This Kiwi-Strawberry Smoothie is a great source of vitamin C, fiber, and potassium. It's also high in protein thanks to the Greek yogurt, making it a good option for a post-workout snack or breakfast. The addition of almond milk provides some healthy fats, while the honey adds a touch of sweetness. Overall, this smoothie is easy to make, delicious, and a great way to start your day or satisfy a sweet craving.

Nutrition Information (per serving):
- Calories: 250
- Protein: 14g
- Carbs: 39g
- Fat: 4g

INGREDIENTS

- 1 cup chopped fresh pineapple
- 1/2 cup coconut milk
- 1/2 cup ice cubes
- 1 tablespoon honey

INSTRUCTIONS

1. Add the chopped pineapple, coconut milk, ice cubes, and honey to a blender.
2. Blend on high speed until the mixture is smooth and creamy.
3. Pour the smoothie into a glass and enjoy immediately.

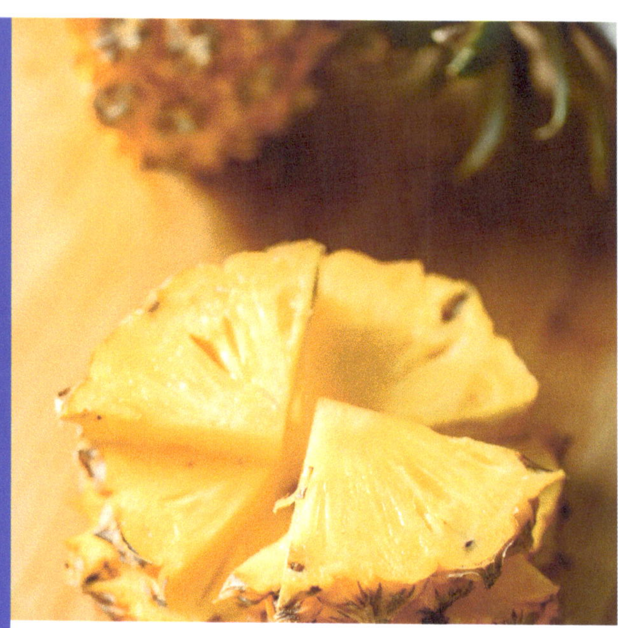

PINEAPPLE-COCONUT SMOOTHIE

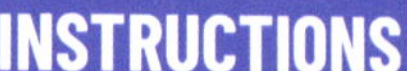 1 servings   5 minutes

This smoothie is a good source of vitamin C, manganese, and copper from the pineapple, which can support immune function, bone health, and energy metabolism. The coconut milk provides healthy fats and a creamy texture while the honey adds natural sweetness. The combination of flavors makes it a delicious tropical treat that can be enjoyed as a healthy snack or breakfast option. This smoothie is easy to make and requires only a few ingredients.

Nutrition Information (per serving):

- Calories: 270
- Protein: 2g
- Carbohydrates: 35g
- Fat: 14g

INGREDIENTS

- 1 small beetroot, peeled and chopped
- 1 cup mixed berries (strawberries, raspberries, blueberries) 1/2 cup
- unsweetened almond milk 1/2 cup plain
- Greek yogurt 1 tbsp honey 1/2 tsp vanilla
- extract
-

INSTRUCTIONS

1. Add the chopped beetroot, mixed berries, almond milk, Greek yogurt, honey, and vanilla extract to a blender.
2. Blend on high until smooth, scraping down the sides as needed.
3. If the mixture is too thick, add more almond milk until you reach the desired consistency.
4. Pour the smoothie into a glass and enjoy immediately.

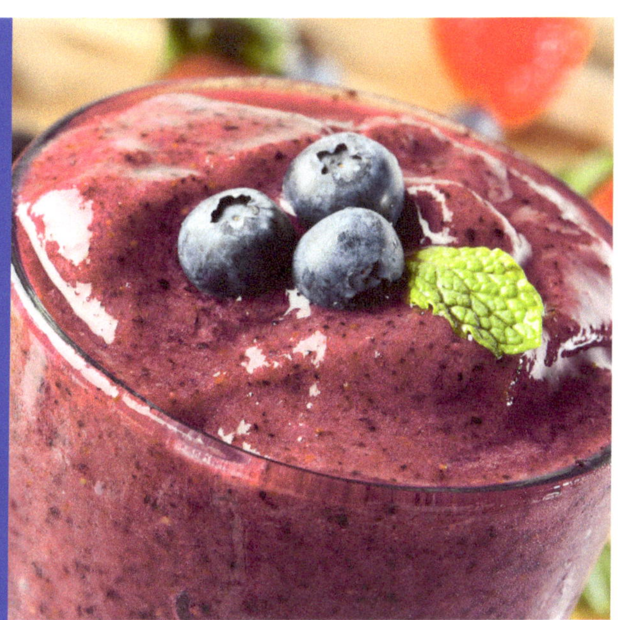

BERRY-BEET SMOOTHIE

🍴 1 servings   🕐 5 minutes

This smoothie is easy to make and offers numerous health benefits. The beetroot in this smoothie provides essential vitamins and minerals, such as folate, potassium, and vitamin C. The mixed berries add a natural sweetness, while also providing antioxidants and fiber. The Greek yogurt offers protein and probiotics, while the almond milk is a great dairy-free alternative. Overall, this smoothie is a delicious and nutritious way to start your day or as a healthy snack.

Nutrition Information (per serving):
• Calories: 310
• Protein: 18g
• Carbohydrates: 49g
• Fat: 4g

- 1 cup spinach
- 1/2 avocado
- 1/2 cucumber
- 1/2 banana
- 1/2 cup almond milk
- 1/4 cup plain Greek yogurt
- 1 tbsp honey
- Juice of 1/2 lime
- 1/2 tsp grated ginger

1. Wash and chop the spinach, avocado, and cucumber into small pieces.
2. Peel and slice the banana.
3. In a blender, combine the spinach, avocado, cucumber, banana, almond milk, Greek yogurt, honey, lime juice, and grated ginger.
4. Blend until smooth and creamy.
5. Pour the smoothie into a glass and enjoy!

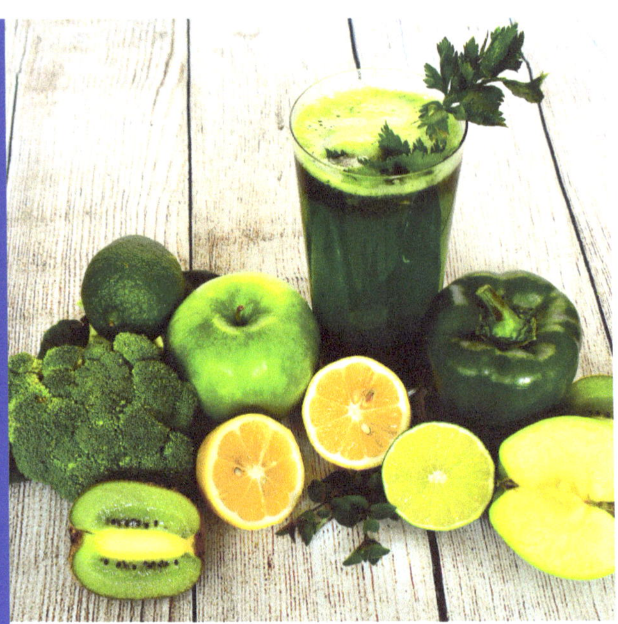

GREEN GODDESS SMOOTHIE

🍴 1 servings   🕐 5 minutes

This smoothie is relatively easy to make, and it's packed with nutrients like potassium, fiber, and healthy fats from avocado. The spinach provides a boost of vitamins A and C, while the cucumber adds a refreshing flavor. The Greek yogurt adds protein and creaminess, while the honey adds sweetness. The ginger and lime juice give a zingy flavor to this delicious smoothie. Overall, this smoothie is an excellent way to start your day with a healthy and tasty breakfast.

Nutrition Information (per serving):
- Calories: 330
- Protein: 8g
- Carbs: 39g
- Fat: 15g

INGREDIENTS

- 1 cup fresh or frozen blackberries
- 1/2 cup unsweetened coconut milk
- 1/2 cup plain Greek yogurt
- 1 tablespoon honey
- 1/2 teaspoon vanilla extract
- 1/2 cup ice cubes

INSTRUCTIONS

1. Add the blackberries, coconut milk, Greek yogurt, honey, and vanilla extract to a blender.
2. Blend on high until smooth and well combined.
3. Add the ice cubes to the blender and blend again until smooth and frothy.
4. Pour the smoothie into a glass and enjoy!

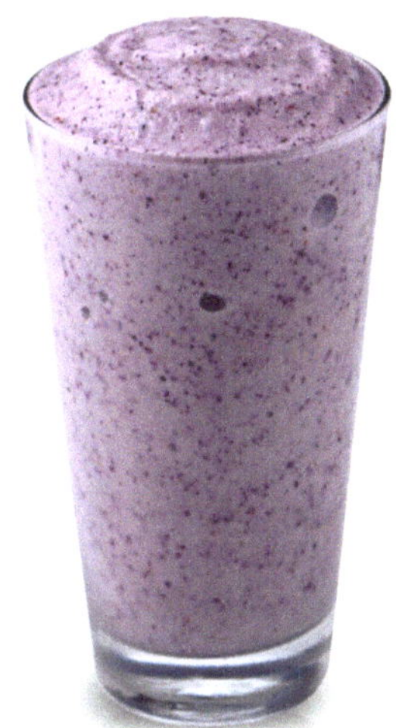

BLACKBERRY-COCONUT SMOOTHIE

 1 servings 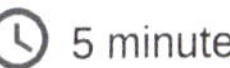 5 minutes

This smoothie is easy to make and packed with flavor. Blackberries are high in antioxidants and vitamin C, while coconut milk adds creaminess and healthy fats. Greek yogurt provides protein and a tangy flavor, while honey and vanilla extract add natural sweetness. Enjoy this smoothie as a tasty and nutritious breakfast or snack.

Nutrition Information (per serving):

- Calories: 350
- Protein: 17g
- Carbs: 41g
- Fat: 7g

INGREDIENTS

- 1 ripe banana
- 1 tablespoon Nutella
- 1/2 cup milk
- 1/2 cup ice cubes
- 1/4 teaspoon vanilla extract
- Optional: whipped cream and chocolate syrup for topping

INSTRUCTIONS

1. Peel the banana and cut it into chunks.
2. In a blender, add the banana chunks, Nutella, milk, ice cubes, and vanilla extract.
3. Blend on high speed until the ingredients are well combined and the mixture is smooth and creamy.
4. Pour the smoothie into a glass.
5. Optional: top with whipped cream and chocolate syrup.

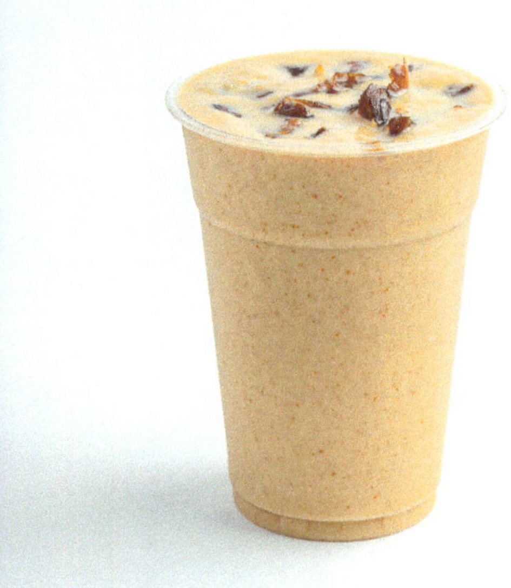

BANANA-NUTELLA SMOOTHIE

🍴 1 servings   🕐 5 minutes

This smoothie is easy to make and offers a delicious, indulgent treat with the creamy banana and chocolate hazelnut flavor of Nutella. Bananas are a good source of potassium and fiber, while Nutella adds a rich and indulgent taste. Milk provides protein and calcium, making this smoothie a filling and satisfying snack or breakfast option.

Nutrition Information (per serving):

- Calories: 370
- Protein: 5g
- Carbs: 50g
- Fat: 13g

INGREDIENTS

- 1 cup frozen raspberries
- 1/2 cup chopped pineapple
- 1/2 cup vanilla Greek yogurt
- 1/4 cup almond milk
- 1 tbsp honey
- 1/4 tsp vanilla extract
- 1/2 cup ice cubes

INSTRUCTIONS

1. In a blender, combine the frozen raspberries, chopped pineapple, vanilla Greek yogurt, almond milk, honey, vanilla extract, and ice cubes.
2. Blend until smooth and creamy, scraping down the sides of the blender as needed.
3. If the smoothie is too thick, add more almond milk until it reaches the desired consistency.
4. Pour the smoothie into a glass and enjoy!

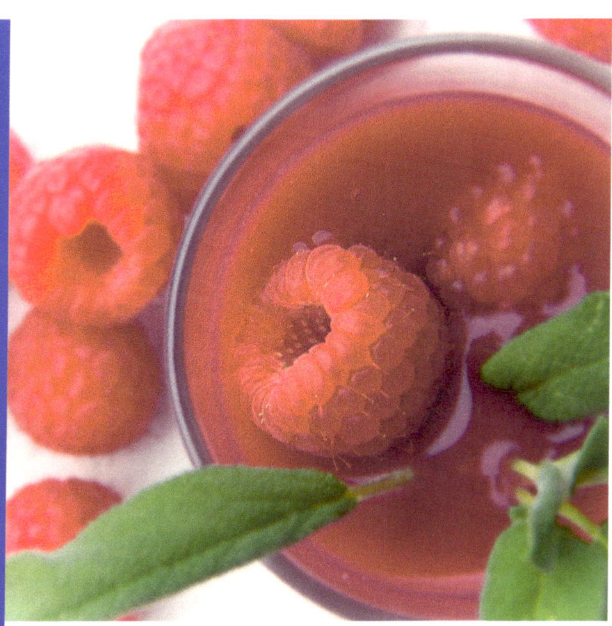

RASPBERRY-PINEAPPLE SMOOTHIE

🍴 1 servings   🕐 5 minutes

This smoothie is easy to make and packed with nutrients. Raspberries and pineapples are both high in vitamin C and antioxidants, which can help boost your immune system and protect against diseases. Greek yogurt provides a good source of protein and probiotics, which can aid in digestion and gut health. Almond milk is a low-calorie and dairy-free alternative to traditional milk, and adds a creamy texture to the smoothie.

Nutrition Information (per serving):
- Calories: 430
- Protein: 16g
- Carbs: 75g
- Fat: 6g

INGREDIENTS

- 1 cup frozen blueberries
- 1 medium-sized peach, peeled and chopped
- 1/2 cup Greek yogurt
- 1/2 cup unsweetened almond milk
- 1 tablespoon honey
- 1/4 teaspoon vanilla extract

INSTRUCTIONS

1. Add all the ingredients into a blender.
2. Blend until smooth and creamy.
3. If the smoothie is too thick, add a little more almond milk until you reach your desired consistency.
4. Pour into a glass and enjoy!

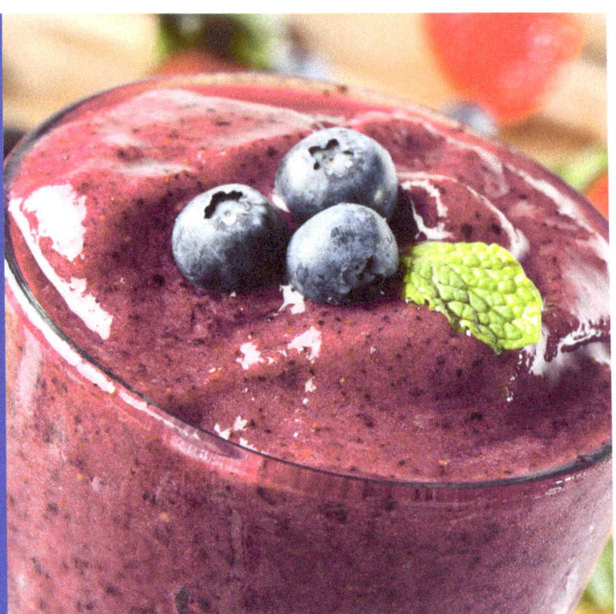

BLUEBERRY-PEACH SMOOTHIE

🍴 1 servings 🕐 5 minutes

This smoothie is very easy to make and is perfect for a quick and healthy breakfast or snack. Blueberries are a great source of antioxidants, while peaches are packed with vitamin C. The Greek yogurt and almond milk provide protein and calcium, making this smoothie a great way to start your day!

Nutrition Information (per serving):
- Calories:450
- Protein: 14g
- Carbs: 60g
- Fat: 7g

- 1 tsp matcha powder
- 1/2 cup unsweetened vanilla almond milk
- 1/2 frozen banana
- 1/2 cup frozen pineapple chunks
- 1/2 tsp honey
- 1/2 tsp vanilla extract
- 1 scoop vanilla protein powder (optional)
- 1/2 cup ice cubes

INSTRUCTIONS

1. In a blender, add the matcha powder and almond milk. Blend until well combined.
2. Add the frozen banana, frozen pineapple chunks, honey, vanilla extract, and protein powder (if using). Blend until smooth.
3. Add the ice cubes and blend until smooth and creamy.
4. Pour the smoothie into a glass and serve.

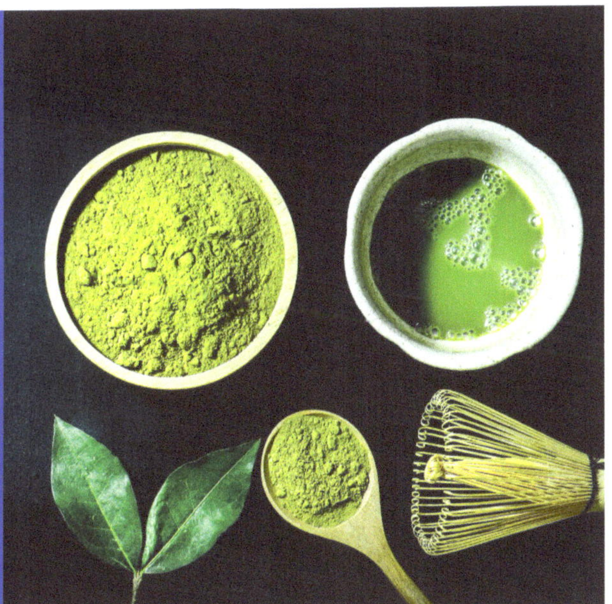

MATCHA-GREEN TEA SMOOTHIE

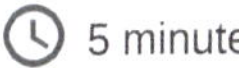 1 servings 🕐 5 minutes

This recipe is easy to make and provides a good source of protein and carbohydrates. Matcha powder is high in antioxidants and can help boost metabolism, while green tea has been linked to numerous health benefits, including improved brain function and lower risk of certain diseases.

Nutrition Information (per serving):

- Calories: 470
- Protein: 20g
- Carbs: 40g
- Fat: 3g

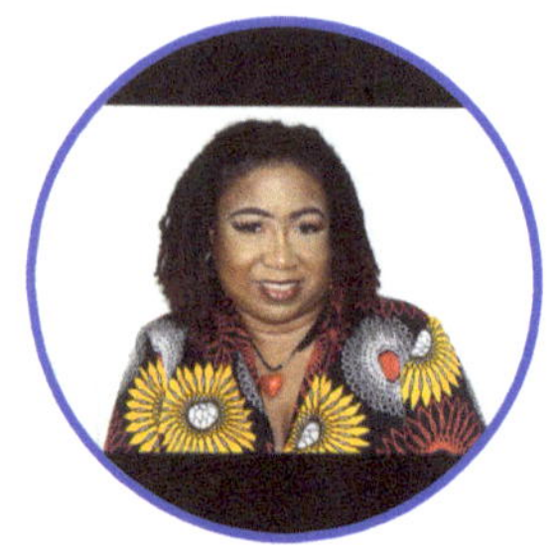

THANK YOU

for making my day so special

Thank You for Purchasing My 28-Day Detox Smoothie eBook!
I want to extend our sincerest gratitude for choosing my 28-Day Detox Smoothie eBook. We hope that this cookbook will help you on your journey to a healthier lifestyle by providing delicious and nutritious smoothie recipes.
My team has put a lot of effort into creating this cookbook, carefully selecting ingredients and testing recipes to ensure that they are not only tasty but also beneficial for your body. We believe that smoothies are an excellent way to boost your health and energy levels, and we hope that our recipes will help you achieve your health goals.
I appreciate your trust in my expertise, and I hope that you will enjoy trying out my smoothie recipes. If you have any questions or feedback, please do not hesitate to contact me. I am always happy to hear from customers and improve our products to meet their needs.
Thank you once again for choosing my 28-Day Detox Smoothie eBook. I wish you all the best on your health journey!
Best regards,

-Dr.Maria

FIND US ON:

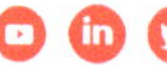

@sonjasecrets
www.sonjasecrets.com